Jane Doe: Gutted.

Prologue

Using the appeal of a novella, Dr. Briones helps us to understand that prevention is a superior medical strategy for Americans. In addition to exercise, natural diets are a critically important dimension of prevention. We are what we eat.

Processed foods with far too many artificial additives and preservatives along with fried foods from fast food restaurants have become part of the staple American diet. Thus, we are becoming toxin loaded obese people. One need only walk through a shopping mall or a large discount store to develop an estimate of the rate of obesity in this country. Our ancestors were leaner than we are today and our ancestors had less toxins in their bodies.

As the U.S. Health Care System increasingly becomes focused on allocating limited health care resources, we have a choice. We can either become more responsible for our own health through prevention, diet and exercise, or we can become increasingly dependent on government decisions concerning allocation of those limited health care resources. Although surgery, especially for the removal of organs, can work miracles, Dr. Briones argues convincingly that we can avoid some surgeries with a lifetime of prevention and a focus on wellness. Otherwise, we might face a future of limited life spans and inability to find health care when needed.

In Jane Doe 2: Gutted, Dr. Briones argues that the misfortune of dementia can be delayed for years with a focus on wellness, exercise and healthy eating. Given the size of the aging baby boom generation, prevention of dementia becomes a larger issue every day.

We should all enjoy the vegetables and fruits from our gardens as we work daily to prevent many avoidable health care issues through diet, exercise and wellness.

Michael J. Stahl, Ph.D.
William B. Stokely Professor of Business
Program Director
Physician Executive MBA Program
College of Business Administration
The University of Tennessee

Jane Doe: Gutted.

Dedication:

To my beloved relative who's appendix I could not save and to my dad who at 73 still has all his organs and his brilliant mind.

Jane Doe: Gutted.

Acknowledgements

Special thanks to Dr. Michael Stahl, Program Director of the Physician Executive MBA program at the University of Tennessee for contributing the prologue and for his leadership in a program that not only taught me how to navigate the troubled waters of health care but how to solve problems by looking at the big picture. My list of achievements since graduating from PEMBA include MDePortal and integrated electronic medical record that can enter data from a smart phone or any device with internet access, a Sleep Disorders Center, a MediSpa, one patent and one patent pending for the use of a technology that will revolutionize the treatment of sleep disorders, a cancer rehab program and functional medicine program that are under development at the time of this publication.

Many thanks as well to all the professors at the American Academy of Antiaging Medicine, in particular Dr. Daniel Amen, whom I call the father of modern psychiatry, for teaching me how to preserve people's organs, specially the brain. Life is so short to accomplish all the goals I have but thanks to what I learned at the American Academy of Antiaging Medicine and at the University of Tennessee PEMBA program I am able to preserve my health and the health of others.

Thanks to my consultants Don Blesdoe and Sean Moran for making this book a reality and to my book cover designer Amanda Struz, award winner not only of Jane Doe: a Cancer Story but for Jane Doe: gutted.

Jane Doe: Gutted.

Preface

This book is one in a series of novellas designed to entertain and educate the public about living healthier lives. "Jane Doe: A Cancer Story," tells the story of an unidentified patient admitted to the Emergency Room who is dying from complications of lung cancer.

"Jane Doe 2: Gutted," tells of the frequent history of women losing their crucial internal organs by the age of 60 and ultimately losing their cognitive functions. Presenting in full Stage 5 dementia, our Jane Doe exemplifies an all-too-common scenario in our emergency rooms across the country.

"Let food be your medicine and medicine be your food."
Hippocrates, 400 B.C.
Father of Modern Medicine

"Behold, I have given you every green plant, and it shall be food for you."
Genesis 1:29

"May you make lots of money and spend it all on doctor bills."
An old Gypsy curse

Death begins in the colon."
Eli Metchnikov, PhD
Nobel Prize in Medicine, 1908

"The doctor of the future will give no medicine, but will interest her or his patient in the care of the human frame, in a proper diet, and in the cause and prevention of disease."
Thomas A. Edison, 1847-1931
U.S. Inventor

"The bacteria is nothing. The terrain is all."
Louis Pasteur 1822-1895
Co-Founder of Microbiology

In good health,

Liam Alexander Briones MD, MBA, FCCP, FSCCM, FAASM, FAAAARM, ABAARM

Jane Doe: Gutted.

Table of Contents

1. The Mall
2. Things Remembered
3. The Good Life
4. A not so good life
5. Sex, Drama, no Rock-n-Roll
6. Meat No More
7. The Inquisition
8. Things Forgot
9. Reunion
10. Evaluation

Jane Doe: Gutted.

Chapter 1 — The Mall

The sad-assed holiday decorations danced and sagged in the cold wind, some of the lights twinkled, but most did not. What was once a vibrant evergreen festooned with pine cones and red ribbons had now faded with time and reflected the age of the mall.

Springfield Mall was the invention of Grover Torkelsen, a local entrepreneur and self-made millionaire who turned a used car lot into the shopping mecca it once was. Formerly anchored by major stores having since moved out, the mall constituted an eclectic collection of mini stores, tired boutiques and a fast food court.

Java Jane's was the go-to place for coffee and donuts, clean and functional, albeit a bit sparse. The coffee was hot, cheap and the donuts, although not made on-site, were brought in fresh every morning.

Doris Finley, a woman in her sixties. Her appearance was clean but not crisp, her manner pleasant but a bit aloof.

As she waited her turn in the short line, her hand fiddled in her overcoat pocket as if she was searching for her change.

"Welcome to Java Jane's. How can I help you?" the overly-made-up teen stated brightly, happy to have her job, "Our donut special today is double-glazed. What can I get you?"

Doris shook her head as if to answer "no." She pulled her hand from her pocket and spilled the contents out on the counter. Among the loose change, much of it pennies, were a myriad of notes.

"Okay, let's see," as she helped Doris with her order.

She separated the notes from the money, picked up today's note and read it to Doris.

"Monday, coffee, shop, gas bill, okay here's some change."

Another note as the clerk noticed the line lengthening.

Jane Doe: Gutted.

"Get money, that's a good one."

She continued to separate the change until she collected enough to buy a cup.

"Just coffee?"

"That would be lovely," Doris nodded.

The clerk served the coffee as Doris scraped together her belongings from the counter and took her coffee to a nearby table. She sat quietly and sipped her coffee as she read over her notes.

After she finished, she pocketed her notes and all the packets of artificial sweetener on the table. No one noticed, but she also took her spoon, overtly slipped into her coat.

Doris wandered out into the near-empty mall, gazing into the windows of the remaining stores still open for business. She stopped abruptly at the display window for "Steven's Apparel, Your Family Clothing Store." In the window, the aging mannequins of a family dressed in winter clothing were posed.

Doris counts the children, "One. Two. Three."

Confused, she recounted slowly, "One. Two. Three"

She pointed to the third child mannequin, tapping loudly on the glass, "Who is the extra child?" She lingered at the window, unsure of what to do next.

Heavenly Detours was one of the successful small boutique stores in the mall that catered to unique moderately-priced gifts.

The one-of-a-kind items were beautifully displayed on pristine glass shelves illuminated by sparkling white twinkle lights. One might think they were placed there for the holiday season, but one would be wrong.

Grace Gallagher, the proprietor, found the lights enchanting, both to the spirit and to the buyer. She relished in catering to both. Grace had been the owner for many years following termination from her job at St.

Jane Doe: Gutted.

Francis Hospital. Most who knew her were shocked, but Grace took it in stride. It was all part of the plan.

Completing the rest of the staff at Heavenly Detours was two of Champlain Valley Union's finest juniors, Heather and Olivia. Earning minimum wage, $7.85, their dedication was dubious. Most of their time was spent sneaking text messages to their school friends and under-ringing totals at the cash register in order to get a little extra on the side. They delighted in the fact they were putting one over on old Grace.

Grace knew it all along. Someone bigger than her would give them a little hell.

Heather's phone alerted her to an incoming text. She turned around from her work.

"It's Ruben," she squealed.

She showed the text to Olivia and her eyes lit up.

"Where is he doing this from?" Olivia inquired.

"The garage, I guess," Heather shrugged.

"I can't believe he's pulled them so far down."

Scrolling to a new picture, Heather indicates, "This is the one from last night."

"OMG. It is huge!" Olivia giggled, as Heather joins in.

The shop bell rang sweetly as the girls were shocked into reality. Heather quickly pocketed her phone and plastered her best fake smile on her face. Oddly, Olivia had the same plastic smile glued to her face as she positioned herself behind the register.

Doris eased into the shop and slowly perused the merchandise as she strolled up and down each aisle. Humming to herself, she was enthralled by all the sparkly goodies. One particular trinket immediately caught her eye.

The snow globe was a beautiful miniature depicting a small country church, complete with a steeple and cross. As she shook it, she

Jane Doe: Gutted.

herself quivered with delight. Without a second thought or looking around, she calmly placed it in her pocket.

Of course, this was not missed by the usually inattentive girls.

Doris smiled as she moved past the girls and up another aisle.

Heather turned to Olivia and silently mouthed, "Do you believe that?"

Doris had stopped, fascinated by another object, which she also pocketed.

Olivia leaned in to Heather, "Go get Grace. We have to call the cops."

Heather, thrilled at the excitement, almost skipped to the back of the shop.

Grace looked up from the inventory sheets.

"Mrs. Gallagher?" Heather asked, "Some old lady out there is shoplifting. We saw it with our own eyes, so we need to call the cops."

Calmly, Grace questioned Heather.

"Are you sure of what you saw, Heather?"

"Absolutely," she adamantly stated.

Grace moved to the front of the shop to size up the situation and found Olivia already on the phone.

As Grace approached Doris, the woman in her sixties turned and smiled.

Grace recognized her instantly and immediately turned to Olivia, saying, "Please hang up the phone."

"But she's stealing right off the shelf," Olivia countered.

"She would never steal, I know her. She's terribly confused."

Grace turned back toward the woman.

"Doris, is there something I can help you with?" Grace was deliberate and calming, her tone reassuring.

Jane Doe: Gutted.

The woman immediately lashed out at Grace, striking her and knocking her down. As Grace fell, she hit her head and shattered one of lower glass shelves as she passed out.

Doris' mood shifted again and she bent down to comfort her victim and cut her hand severely.

Heather screamed to Olivia, "Call 911 right away."

St. Francis Memorial Hospital was one of those turn of the century hospitals updated to a modern facility now held by a large Catholic conglomerate. The facility boasts the latest, cutting-edge medical technology and professionals. It also boasted the last remaining emergency room facility within fifty miles.

Christmas time in the E.R. was as festive as hell. Out came every lunatic case along with real emergencies. Waiting to be seen in the E.R. was a sampling of the homeless, most with frostbite, a young boy burned from a stove accident and several elderly patients. The most serious had severe chest pains and was being treated in one of the bays.

Presiding over this mayhem was Chip "Hotshot" Fitzgerald, fresh from med school, top of his class and beautifully tanned. The nurses imagined he perfected his tan sunning on the beach in a very small Speedo with them. Unbeknownst to them, he was gay and shacked up with a younger man even hotter than himself.

His right-hand was Nurse Connie Rossi, a full-figured woman with an infectious laugh. Her mantra was "I'll give you the shirt off my back, but be ready to meet the girls." Hotshot adored her.

Also on the shift were a handful of dedicated nurses doing their best to make things flow. The only wrench in the machinery was Darren Eammon, a first year resident whose attitude was bigger than his privates. In a collaborative world like the E.R., me-centric people don't fit in. Hello, Dr. Eammon.

"Unit 5," the radio spit.

"Copy," Connie grabbed the mic.

Jane Doe: Gutted.

"Inbound, female, sixties, severe lacerations to both hands, stable but disoriented, ETA five minutes," came the reply.

Connie turned to alert Dr. Fitzgerald, but was interrupted.

"Unit 2."

"Copy."

"Same incident, second female, seventies, head trauma, stable and responding to commands, ETA five minutes."

Connie momentarily leaves her station and found Dr. Fitzgerald flirting as usual with another nurse.

"Put down the cookie, it'll ruin your figure," Connie said, "Like that'll ever happen. We've got a couple incoming."

Connie continued to brief Dr. Fitzgerald as nurse Watkins and Hernandez, the lone male nurse on the shift, gloved up.

Dr. Fitzgerald turned toward the nurses, "Where the hell is Eammon?"

"Check the men's room. 'Mirror, mirror, on the wall,'" Hernandez quipped.

Red lights flashed around the waiting room.

"Go get him," Fitzgerald said and then turned to nurse Watkins, "Linda, come with me."

They head to the entrance to intercept the EMTs with the first patient as they rolled her in.

The EMT apprised Fitzgerald.

"We've stabilized her, but she's lost a lot of blood. She's confused and appears to be extremely disoriented."

"Do we know her name?"

"A Jane Doe, non-responsive."

"Get her into bay number two."

As Watkins heads off with the EMTs to assist in the patient transfer, Fitzgerald stops Eammon on his way out.

Jane Doe: Gutted.

"You need to be on the floor. Take your potty breaks later," he snapped.

Eammon's sour face mumbled something under his breath.

"My E.R., my rules," Fitzgerald smiled firmly.

Eammon and Hernandez intercepted the second gurney.

Grace Gallagher knew this E.R. like the back of her hand, although it had the freshness of new paint and equipment, she had worked in these halls for years.

Jane Doe: Gutted.

Chapter 2 — Things Remembered

Athens, Ohio in the early fifties was booming with Eichler-esque affordable tract houses for the families of the returning veterans from World War II. Joseph Eichler was known for his developments in California after the war and many cities copied his success. Little houses with little lawns and little backyards and landscaping. All the houses looked alike and in those days no one locked their doors. Many an inebriated husband found himself in a neighbor's living room by mistake.

At 188 Tracey Drive, the home of Ralph and Emma Finley was in the midst of breakfast and the get to work and school routine. Jimmy, 9, and Louise, 7, were fighting over the last of the milk, as usual, for their corn flakes.

"You're using too much milk," Louise exclaimed, as Jimmy poured from the glass bottle.

"Jimmy, share with your sister and sit down," Emma pleaded as she juggled her husband's breakfast and the whining baby Doris in her arms.

"I'm just barely covering the corn flakes," Jimmy retorted.

"Cover them less and pass the bottle to Louise."

She set her husband's place at the table and worked diligently to appease the baby.

"C'mon sweetheart, why are you still crying? Are you hungry? Are you thirsty." She felt the cotton diaper. "You're not wet."

Her blue-collar husband, Ralph, never a morning person, seemed a bit gruffer than usual as he let loose a burp to the amusement of the children.

"Ralph, please," Emma gently chastised.

"What. It's just natural," as he planted himself at the table. "What's wrong with her now?" he nodded toward the baby.

Jane Doe: Gutted.

"She's been like this all night," Emma sighed heavily, "I may have to take her to the doctor."

"Shit," he mumbled under his breath.

Emma gave her husband "the look." She knew the budget was tight, she did the shopping, the cooking, sewed the clothes and cut corners where she could. Ralph's factory salary was barely covering a family of four so when Doris arrived, things got even tighter.

It strained the budget and their relationship.

"Maybe she's just a whiny kid, Jimmy was."

"Was not," Jimmy interrupted with his mouth full.

"You sure were. Cried all the time. And quit talkin' with your mouth full."

Ralph accusingly turned to Emma, "Why does it always have to be the doctor?"

"Something's wrong, I just know it."

Ralph muttered as he quickly finished his breakfast, stood up and polished off his coffee.

"Have a good day at work," as she tried half-heartedly to put a smile on her face as the door slammed closed.

"Okay, kids, finish up so you can get ready for school," she said, exasperated.

"But mom, there's no school, it's Saturday," Jimmy whined.

Emma sighed heavily as she eased into a chair at the table.

"I've just lost track of the time."

Children in tow, dressed for the day, Emma and the kids waited for the city bus at the stop two blocks from the house. The kids were fidgeting with excitement at the prospect of riding the bus around town.

"When we get on the bus, you sit quietly and behave," she warned. "I've got enough to handle with your sister."

The bus noisily arrived at the stop and they all boarded. Once underway, the baby cried more loudly, irritating the other passengers.

Jane Doe: Gutted.

Emma tried unsuccessfully to quiet the child and was nearly at her wits end.

The stop for Main Street and Dr. Hall's office was next.

"Jimmy, stand up and pull the cord."

Excitedly, he pulled the cord and the bus stopped at the next stop, where they discharged onto the curb. Emma sighed in relief as she escaped from the looks from the other passengers who seemed relieved to see them go.

Emma and the kids walked up the block to the doctor's office, and enjoyed the warmth of a nice spring day.

As they climbed the steps to the office, Emma's face registered disappointment as she read the hand-scrawled note cellophane taped to the door: "Vacation day, for emergencies go to St. Francis." She tried to hold on to what little patience she had left.

She looked around to get her bearings and handed the baby to Jimmy.

"Why do I get her? I'm a boy. Dad never holds the baby," he protested.

"You're nine. You can help me out here," as she opened her pocketbook. She looked in, pulled out her change purse and peered inside. With a snap, she closed it and she thrust it back into her pocketbook.

"We'll walk."

They trudged up the hill the four blocks to the emergency room.

St. Francis resembled a medieval fortress, brick and stone. It consisted of the main building of eight floors built in the early 1900s with a newer addition added in the late-forties. The hospital was operated by the Sisters of Mercy, a Catholic order founded in Ireland by Catherine McAuley.

Jane Doe: Gutted.

Stepping into the emergency room, the first thing Emma noticed was that unique odor of dried blood, saliva and alcohol. Layered over that was the odd disinfectant they all used which rarely worked.

"It smells in here!" Jimmy exclaimed as he held his nose.

"Jimmy, take your sister over to those chairs and wait for me," Emma said.

Waiting for the inevitable was a big a part of the E.R. from its inception. The procedure for wait times depended on the acuity of the patients at any given day. Depending on the severity of your illness you would be triaged at a lower level than a heart attack or serious injury.

"Good morning, Sister..." Emma read her nametag, "Mary Luke."

A pleasantly plump nun clad in a white nursing habit smiled at Emma through her thick coke bottle glasses.

"How may I help you this morning, dear?"

"My baby Doris has been sick for the last couple of days and I know something is not right. I went to the doctor's office and a note on the door said to come here," Emma related.

"Help me narrow this down a bit for the form. Throat? Eyes? Ears? Any of those?" the Sister asked and Emma shook her head.

"It seems to be her stomach," she replied.

"Any vomiting or diarrhea?"

"A bit of both," Emma hesitated to say.

"Blood?"

"I don't believe so," Emma affirmed.

Sister Mary Luke made a few notes and turned the paper toward Emma.

"Please sign here and take a seat."

As Emma signed the papers, Sister Mary Luke surveyed the waiting room. In the room were several waiting patients including an elderly man and a middle-aged woman who appeared to be extremely pale.

Jane Doe: Gutted.

"From what I see here, your wait should be short," and she leaned into Emma, "Sit away from the lady in the blue coat, we're not sure what she has." Emma looked over her shoulder, moved to sit as far away from the blue lady as possible and motioned for the kids to join her. Jimmy and Louise had been standing at the window watching the cars.

Then Doris began to wail loudly. Once again, Emma endured the intense stares from those nearby, including the lady in blue from across the room.

Sister Mary Luke walked over to Emma.

"Mrs. Finley, we're ready for you and the baby now," she then noticed the other kids, "On second thought, you'd better bring everyone."

Emma was ushered into an examination room. From the looks on the faces of the children, the circus had just come to town. Before them was a huge array of bizarre equipment that gleamed, beeped and blinked. To one side, the suture tray had really captivated Jimmy's attention. It contained the needle holders, the forceps, the scissors and various small bowls and sterile towels. Louise stood in awe of the orthopedic equipment, complete with shoulder slings and cervical collars which she immediately began to try on.

"Louise, put that down, please," Emma urged as Doris continued to wail, tugging at the last thread of patience she had left.

"Don't worry, she can't hurt anything. You go ahead. You can be my helper for this examination," said a handsome, slightly-balding, middle-aged doctor who appeared at the door and walked in to greet Emma, "Also helping today is Nurse Gallagher, but we all call her Grace."

Next to enter was a beautiful, young nurse. She was well coiffed and starched from her white polished shoes to the cap on her head.

"Let me take Doris," Grace said.

Once the baby was in the arms of the nurse, she fell silent.

"I could sure use you at home," Emma sighed.

Jane Doe: Gutted.

The doctor laughed, "Grace has that calming effect on most people. That's why we keep her around even though she's not a nun."

"Shall I undress her Dr. Casey?" Grace asked.

"Please," Dr. Dan Casey replied as he turned to Emma, who was keeping an eye on Jimmy and Louise.

"Those two will be fine, so tell me about Doris," he asked.

As Grace readies Doris for the examination, Dr. Casey listened intently to the symptoms listed by Emma.

"Well, I share your concern and there are number of possibilities," he said.

Louise wandered over and pulled the stethoscope from his pocket. As he continued to speak to Emma, he put the stethoscope to her ears and showed her how to listen to her heart.

"My first inclination is a urinary tract infection or gastritis. The other ailments are a bit more serious."

"And they would be?" Emma gulped.

"Gall bladder problems or appendicitis, but let's just take a look."

Dr. Casey rose and walked to the examination table where Grace waited with baby Doris. As he examined the baby, he explained his procedure while performing it.

"The first procedure we'll do is an abdominal exam to detect inflammation. If we find none, then there are urine and blood tests to determine the problem. No sooner had he uttered the words, he gently prodded the stomach and Doris screamed instantly. Not having a poker face, he winced slightly at the sound.

"That's not good, is it?" Emma queried.

Uncharacteristically for a nurse, Grace chimed in, "There are still the other tests we can do. Don't jump to conclusions just yet."

Dr. Casey's face expressed the same disdain at Grace's opinion as it did Doris' scream. He turned to Grace.

"Please get a blood and urine sample from the child," he scolded.

Jane Doe: Gutted.

Realizing no mother ever wanted to see their small child enduring a medical exam, he ushered her to the small desk in the corner of the examination room. In his mind, he already knew it was appendicitis. He would follow the standard procedure and perform an appendectomy.

As Grace struggled with Doris to extract her blood, the more difficult task was the next step, getting the urine sample. Getting a toddler to pee on command is nearly impossible.

As Grace continued with the patient, she kept an ear open to the conversation between Dr. Casey and Emma Finley. What was being discussed was of great concern to Grace. She was afraid that traditional medicine and "standard procedures" often led women down a dangerous path. In her ultimate wisdom, she knew more than the doctors. She also knew there were alternatives to the last remaining option — surgery. The problem was that Grace was the nurse, not the doctor.

"Most of us think the appendix is a vestigial organ," Dr. Casey explained as Emma shook her head, completely lost, "That simply means we feel it is an organ left over from early man and serves no purpose in the body."

He turned to Grace at the sound of her quiet sigh. He thought it might have been trouble with the patient, but with her stare, he realized the response was from what he had said.

He turned back to Emma and continued, "There are those who think this is not the case," he emphasized with a slight glance over his shoulder, "But they are a small minority outside of the AMA community." He punctuated his statement with a small stamp of his foot. "We are not sure of the cause of appendicitis, but lodged so close to the large intestine, it often becomes clogged with stool and bacteria and becomes inflamed and infected," he paused.

"It needs to come out," he asserted.

Jane Doe: Gutted.

"If untreated, the appendix can burst and your child could die," and before he could continue, Grace dropped the scissors from the exam table.

"I'm so sorry, doctor, they slipped."

He highly doubted her.

"I'm going to give you some antibiotics to slow down the infection in the appendix, but mind you, this is not the cure. It just buys us a little time until we can get the tests back from the lab. It's Saturday, so it will take a little longer than usual, but I will call you by Monday morning at the latest."

Emma gathered up her belongings and took the prescription slip from Dr. Casey.

"Take that slip to Sister Mary Luke and she will give you enough medicine to get through Monday," he finished.

As Dr. Casey made his final notes on Doris Finley's chart, Emma motioned to Jimmy and Louise that they were leaving. She crossed to Grace as Doris was now redressed. With a slight smile, she handed the toddler back to Emma and whispered, "She'll be fine."

"I'll show you back to the waiting area," Grace said as Dr. Casey continued his notes. Little did Dr. Casey realize, he would only be the first of many doctors to add their notes to Doris Finley's chart, which would eventually grow to encompass hundreds of pages.

Grace escorted Emma to the waiting room and noted that it looked like a busy day ahead for the E.R.

"I thought it was going to be a light day, but I could be wrong," said Sister Mary Luke.

"We'll fit them all in, we've seen busier days," Grace smiled as she looked over charts of patients waiting to be seen.

Back in his office, Dr. Casey pondered how he would approach Nurse Grace. Although her work was superb, being attentive to both the

Jane Doe: Gutted.

patient and their needs. It was the attitude she projected during Miss Finley's examination that couldn't be tolerated.

Grace checked her watch, a simple Speidel, a gift from her father on the occasion of receiving the graduation cap from nursing school. The day had passed quickly and she could not remember even pausing for lunch.

Dr. Casey poked his head out from his office, "Miss Gallagher, would you come see me before you clock out, please?"

"Absolutely, doctor," she replied.

Miss Gallagher? She knew this was coming. After finishing her last chart, she helped Sister Mary Luke tidy up the station.

"What did you do now?" she asked knowingly, "Doctor Casey was sure clinical today."

"Silently offered an opinion that wasn't well received," she sighed.

"Is it ever?"

They both smile.

Grace takes a moment in the ladies room to freshen her lipstick, adjust her cap and smooth her uniform. Every little bit helped.

She knocked softly on Dr. Casey's door.

"Come in, please," Dr. Casey said.

Dr. Casey sat behind a large wooden desk with bookcases of medical reference books behind him, his medical diploma from the Cincinnati College of Medicine and specialty certifications hung in large frames on the wall.

"Have a seat," he said, choosing his words carefully. "We have been down this road before," he continued. "Your work is exemplary, but at times your attitude puzzles me. Is there something I don't know?" he pondered.

Grace thought to herself. Oh God, can I please tell him the truth? She remained silent.

Jane Doe: Gutted.

"This morning, we had the case of Doris Finley, a four year old white female, exhibiting classic symptoms of appendicitis. I am sure when we see the blood and urine tests, it will confirm my diagnosis and precipitate an appendectomy procedure."

Grace shifted uncomfortably.

"You obviously do not agree, but this is not medicine by consensus. I am the doctor here. As I said before, I admire your work, but be aware of your position. If it continues, it will be reflected in your personnel file."

Grace bit her lower lip pensively.

"Understood?"

"Yes, doctor."

"That is all for now. Have a good evening."

Reflection

As I lay here on the examination table waiting to be seen, I can tell from the blood flow that the cut on my head is no deeper than one-half inch and a half-dozen butterfly sutures should do the trick. It helps having been a nurse, albeit so long ago. Although the curtain between us is drawn, I can hear them working on Doris in the next bay.

She's had such a long journey to get here from the first day we met fifty-nine years ago. Do you remember me, Doris? I was the one who tried to save you from that appendectomy when you were a child. I got into so much trouble over that. I wanted to tell your Doctor What's-His-Name to give you and your appendix a chance. It is a marvelously useful organ in creating its own probiotics that the body needs. We know now, people without an appendix have an increased risk of colon cancer.

Jane Doe: Gutted.

Now granted, you exhibited abdominal pains, but it could have been many things. Something you ate. Gas. Simple constipation. But no, let's just cut it out. They were so antiquated back then and, at times they often are, but the tides are slowly changing. With better diet, more fruits and vegetables, we can train the gut to be healthier.

Probiotics are the small organisms that help maintain a balance in the intestines. It could be as simple as eating the yogurt that the famous actress promotes on TV.

Then there's glutamine, an amino acid that helps protect the lining of the gastro-intestinal tract.

I need to tell them who you are, Doris Finley. By all appearances, you're in the final stages of dementia and I can't help but wish we could have schooled you in healthier choices for your body. Surgery has its place and many times a miraculous event, but how I wish there had been an alternative outcome for you.

Jane Doe: Gutted.

Chapter Three — The Good Life

A 1975 wedding was everything you thought it would be. Polyester meets disco with a veneer of lace.

Doris Finley and Stefano Costa met in college during a war protest and from all appearances it was love at first sight. The loud noise of the crowd suddenly ceased when Doris laid her eyes on the tall, tan, fit freshman who waved an American Flag several people behind her. It seemed his face glowed when he turned his eyes to her. No doubt an instant Dopamine high. After that they spent every possible moment together, culminating in a midnight picnic on the park reservation complete with wine and cheese. Stefano brought his guitar and serenaded Doris into her first true romance. He was tender, patient and made her feel as though it was his first time, too. The reputation of Italian men was certainly true. Doris had played the part of the shy virgin with several cautionary "no's" but when Stefano disrobed in the moonlight, there before her stood Adonis. Doris blushed as she realized the statues didn't do a particular part justice. Luckily, no park rangers happened by.

Stefano was a second generation Italian man of Sicilian descent. Although with him came all of the joys and trappings of the large Italian family, as Doris was embraced immediately as part of that family.

Doris' own family had tragically shrunk with the passing of her father, Ralph, in a factory accident and the loss of her brother, Jimmy, in Vietnam. Her sister, Louise, had married and her mother, Emma, now worked at St. Francis Memorial in administration.

After the ceremony, lavish for a small city wedding and paid for by the Costa's, Doris and Stefano settled not far from his parents. With the birth of their first child just ten months after their wedding, Doris had

Jane Doe: Gutted.

taken her dutiful place in the family tree. Ricci Stefano was a healthy baby boy and as the first grandson, was heralded king.

Stefano shared in the glory of producing the first grandchild. Except for Stefano's father, Georgio, no one in the family knew was actually his second child. Be it the times or lack of parental guidance about contraception led him to father a baby while exploring sex with a classmate in high school resulted in a baby. Georgio paid the family off and the infant was given up for adoption. Since the secret would have killed Georgio's wife, Sophia, it was taken to his grave.

It would join several of the unspoken events father and son shared. Georgio had fathered several children before his marriage to Sophia and one after. Athens, Ohio was simply too small a city for Stefano not to have met several of his secret siblings. When he confronted his father with questions, they were simply answered, "A man has urges."

Stefano understood this completely. He had been having an affair since the birth of his first child.

Jane Doe: Gutted.

Chapter 4 — A Not So Good Life

Although Stefano understood, a man "having urges," his religious guilt unnerved him. He was not a bad man, but felt like one every time he cheated on Doris. The stress of a young child, an unfulfilling job, an overbearing family and a now-pregnant wife seemed to have thrust him to escape to another woman. Laughingly, he thought how easy it would have been to escape to a man, but he wasn't wired that way.

Doris' second child, Marci, was seemingly born without complications. These would ensue shortly after the child arrived home. In the 70s, little was known about postpartum depression (PPD) or its less-severe version, the "baby blues." One in five mothers were affected and if the depression remained untreated, the mother risked drug and alcohol abuse and in severe cases, suicide.

In Doris' case, her heavy bleeding and poor libido had contributed to the disintegration of their relationship at such an early stage in their marriage.

Dr. Marjorie Van Cleef, was one of the first women gynecologists in the field. Doris had done her research and thought a woman would be more sensitive to her needs. She was incorrect in her assumption, for much like the times, Dr. Van Cleef decided a hysterectomy was the only option and referred Doris to a surgeon at St. Francis.

The surgeon, Dr. Thomas Hastings, had performed this procedure many times and was considered to be one of the best at it. Assisting him was Nurse Grace, now reaching middle age and still of the same opinion that women were still not given non-surgical options. It never even entered into the discussion.

Removing the uterus is an extremely difficult decision in any woman's life. With a hysterectomy, the woman loses her ability to become pregnant, the vagina shortens and some adjustments might need

Jane Doe: Gutted.

to be made during intercourse. Most women are able to still reach orgasm depending on the reason for the hysterectomy. Hormones need to be optimized, however, to make sure the sensitivity of the tissues remains and the mood is optimal for romance. When hysterectomy is performed for heavy bleeding the cause (low progesterone) is not addressed. Progesterone is a calming hormone, achieving orgasm with an anxious mind is very difficult. When progesterone is low, other hormones could be out of balance. So it is important to have the female symphony of hormones optimized not only for preservation of sexual function but for optimization of mood, brain function, bone and muscle integrity that is lost during the aging process. Along with associated risks like blood clots, removal may also damage other nearby organs.

Nurse Grace was able to review Mrs. Costa's chart before seeing her patient. She was anxious to see how, Doris, the child she met twenty-five years earlier, had developed into a young woman. She was saddened at the circumstances of yet another opportunity for medicine to revert to the last stage option, surgery.

"Good morning, Mrs. Costa," Grace said as she entered the room, "Dr. Hastings will be with you shortly."

"Thank you," Doris replied quietly.

Grace had no expectation that Doris would remember her from all those years before, but it was lovely to see that her patient had grown into a lovely woman.

"How are you feeling today?" Grace inquired.

"Fine, under the circumstances."

"I see in your chart you were referred from a Dr. Van Cleef to consult in a possible hysterectomy procedure." Grace said hesitantly.

Doris noticed the tone in Grace's voice.

"It doesn't sound like you're in agreement with the diagnosis."

Grace smiled knowing that saying anything once again will get her another reprimand and possible suspension.

Jane Doe: Gutted.

"Go ahead, I won't tell," she joked.

"Well, I'm not the doctor," she stated.

"Understood," Doris nodded.

She leaned in and whispered, "Has anyone mentioned progesterone?"

Doris shook her head, no.

"It's a supplement. It helps your ovaries, who normally produce this by themselves," Grace pushed on, "With the removal of the uterus, the ovaries normally die within three years."

Doris looked worried and Grace felt guilty.

It was Grace's intent only to educate and not to further depress Doris. She felt women were not given the options.

Both women were startled when Dr. Hastings strode into the room and sensed their conversation. He was troubled and looked directly at Grace.

"Good morning, doctor," Grace said.

"Good morning, Nurse Gallagher," he replied flatly. He turned on the charm and a smile appeared as he turned to Doris.

The charm was part of the bedside manner for a surgeon. Dr. Hastings was a surgeon of the highest caliber and there for one purpose only, surgery — removal of the problem. Sadly for the patient, not many alternatives were offered. In all fairness, surgery was a miracle, but Grace, all-knowing, lived for an educated public and alternatives were part of that education.

Unfortunately for Doris, Grace's suggestion went unheeded and a radical hysterectomy was performed. Yet another step in the gutting of Doris Costa. The surgery harmed her brain by depriving it from much needed good estrogens and not replacing the already missing progesterone and testosterone. The mental fog that women feel during menopause is not a myth.

It is a lack of hormones!

Jane Doe: Gutted.

Jane Doe: Gutted.

Chapter 5 — Sex, Drama, No Rock-n-Roll

A non-event for the Costa's was about to become part of the family tree. Divorce. Georgio and Sophia, Doris' in-laws, had been married for forty-five years and by all outward appearances had the perfect marriage. Obviously, Stefano knew differently. In his mind, divorce was the only out and those, indeed, were the papers served on Doris. The once "golden girl" of the Costa Family was now outcast as the cause of the ruination of the family. Being Italian Catholics, Mama Costa was sure the Pope himself would be contacting the family within the week.

As everyone is a relationship knows, the saying proved true, "it takes two to tango." And tango they did, but not with each other!

As good-looking a man as Stefano certainly was, he had the world at his feet in the dating game of the early 80s. It wasn't exactly free-love of the hippie era, but both reveled in their new-found freedom. The revolving door of Stefano's bachelor digs were an amusement to the building concierge. At first he questioned the "guests" as to who they were visiting, but eventually recognized the type. There were a few he missed. Those were two of the men he presumed to be Stefano's drinking buddies. In fact, they constituted Stefano's dalliances into the world of bisexuality.

On the other hand, Doris' world was far more complex. Now having to raise two children on her own, now finding employment was her number one concern.

Law school was where she found comfort in the pleasant words of her criminal law professor, Anthony Luciano, a distinguished Polish-Italian law professor. This high powered criminal law attorney had taken out the Cleveland mafia back in the 70s. Now, in his mid-50s, was teaching in the Law School at the University of Athens. He also continued to practice for a high profile law firm in town. His six foot

Jane Doe: Gutted.

frame dressed in a three-piece suit with shiny black shoes, pipe in-hand, commanded a presence. Even though balding and not in perfect shape, she enjoyed listening to his deep, firm authoritative voice during class. The polar opposite of Stefano, he was much more comforting. Their cafeteria lunches turned into picnics in the metro parks, but ever the gentleman and aware of his position as her professor, Tony never made a move on Doris. After a year of this "relationship," Doris wondered if Tony was impotent, married or gay. He never spoke of a family or if he even had one. She finally decided to make a move since she had grown fond of him and could think of little else.

"Tony, I have something for you" she said when he answered the phone.

"Sure, I can pick it up after class," he replied, perplexed at the whisper in Doris' voice.

"But I do not want you to read it in front of me or around anybody else. You need to promise me you will read it in private."

Doris had no idea how he would react to the confession of her feelings toward him. She thought of two possible outcomes. Either she would be asked to leave his class or he would simply ignore her. She dared not believe in the third outcome, that he would share her feelings!

Tony finished his class as usual and gingerly approached Doris. He wondered what the big mystery was.

"What is the matter dear?" he asked.

Doris handed him her PalmPC.

"Please do not watch this until you are alone," she pleaded.

Tony's curiosity turned to caution. What would he find? Wondering what he would find, a few thoughts crossed his mind. Instead of going to lunch, he immediately went to his office and opened the device. A power point presentation popped up:

"If you ever feel lonely,

"I am head over heels for you."

Jane Doe: Gutted.

Tony was shaken up. As a professor at the university, befriending a student was allowed, but a sexual relationship was taboo.

He would lose his job in an instant.

Hours passed and Tony was not answering. Doris decided to find out the verdict over the phone, as she could not handle another rejection in person.

"Doris, please understand my position. As a faculty member, I signed a contract that prevents me from having romantic relations with any student. I know you are older than the other students and perfectly capable of making your own decisions but it would be an ethical nightmare for me. You can retrieve your Palm when I see you in class. Good-bye, Doris," said Tony in a kind but firm voice.

Doris hung up the phone and her heart felt heavier than she could bear. When she arrived home, Doris collapsed in tears until she had cried herself to sleep.

He will never speak to me again. What an idiot I was to think any differently. He is a proper, ethical attorney.

The next day at school, Doris sat at the back of the room and for a week it appeared as if Tony was ignoring her.

"Ms. Finley, could you please tell us what are the elements of a first degree murder crime?" he asked.

Doris was caught by surprise and stunned by his aloofness, she answered as best as she could.

At least he didn't kick me out of his class.

After a month of distance, Tony's secretary called Doris, "Mr. Luciano wants to meet you at his law office at noon today at five sixteen Main Street, suite two."

"Oh my God," Doris wondered out loud. Now he's going to reprimand me.

"Sir, Miss Finley is here," the secretary eyed her as she waited.

"Please have her come in," the voice intoned deeply.

Jane Doe: Gutted.

Doris entered an impressive office with a massive antique wooden desk, attorney's ink pens and reference books perfectly aligned on the shelves. In front of a deep cranberry leather sofa, a coffee table was set for lunch, complete with linen table cloth and a bottle of wine in a silver ice bucket. Accompanying this was a serving dish of gourmet hors d'oeuvres with a set of disposable dishes and forks. To top it all off, chocolate dipped strawberries and a red rose bouquet adorned the matching side table. The table lamps were dimmed and the curtains of his rise corner office were closed shut. The atmosphere felt warm and comfortable and completely opposite to the caustic visit with him at school.

Doris heart pounded.

Here she was feeling like a young woman again, this time with a man 18 years her senior. She cleared her throat and wondered if the man behind the desk could hear the pounding in her heart.

He was deeply focused on his current high profile criminal case, the defense of a baby food conglomerate and the alleged death of 11 infants that had consumed the food.

"A settlement is all we'll get here," he thought as he closed the file and raised his eyes to Doris.

His face softened and his eyes sparkled.

"Please have a seat," as he indicated the leather sofa.

Doris sat at the corner of the leather couch as Tony took the seat next to her. Tony sat next to her as if the last month never happened.

Doris' body reacted to his closeness, not out of contempt, but surprise. His reaction was to pull back a bit and adjust at a slight distance.

The conversation was light, like the good old days. He finally opened up and told her of his wife. She had left him for her relationship with another woman and their divorce was almost final. She could barely hear him over her own thoughts.

Jane Doe: Gutted.

"So, what are we doing here?" she thought, "the strawberries, the roses, the wine? Who are they for?" Maybe he has an appointment with a girlfriend later.

Seemingly they were not for someone else because after eating some hors d'oeuvres and enjoying a bit of the wine, the secretary's voice intruded.

"Sir, you need to leave for your class at the University."

"I'm sorry, Doris, I need to go," he said softly.

And gently, he kissed her on the lips.

"I'll be back after class. Please Join me for dessert and flowers."

Doris' heart was coming out of her chest as she left his office. She, too, had to get to the University for the same class.

"What do I do now?" she whispered to herself.

Does this mean we are dating? Is he going get fired? Am I going to get kicked out of law school?

She felt terrified yet could not help wanting to jump up and down with excitement.

As it turned out, this was the beginning of years of intense hidden romance. Doris finally found true love and adventure. They made love with each other intensely in his office and in the parks protected by the darkness of the night. Anywhere. No one could destroy their love. Doris wanted to raise the kids on her own and did not want another man to replace the kids' father, so they had to conceal their love for many but wonderful years.

The final equalizer, death, was the only thing to end the fairy tale relationship. Anthony Luciano died of a massive coronary on the ski slopes of Vail, one of their only vacations away from Athens.

The depression of a loss of life and love was devastating for Doris. People around her who had no idea of the secret relationship, chalked up her catatonic existence as health issues. But, for the living, life goes on, and after a period of private mourning, Doris began to date again. It

Jane Doe: Gutted.

wasn't all sex, although there was plenty, it was what single people did. Also, it was many free dinners for her and helped to supplement the budget of a single mother, as she juggled kids and law school.

Doris' mother, Emma, had hoped she would make time to find someone. After all, she was approaching forty and the clock was ticking. She also felt that Ricci and Marci needed a father. A real father and not a cheater. She never knew if her daughter realized that Stefano had other children with other women, but mother knew all because she worked in records at St. Francis.

She had also befriended a wonderful nurse at the hospital, Grace Gallagher. It started simply as someone to eat lunch with, but blossomed into a true friendship. Emma enjoyed Grace's view of the world, although rather progressive. Nurse Gallagher was constantly on report due to her opinions, often shared with the doctor she worked for. Grace seemingly never realized her position as a nurse was not thought of as a colleague by the doctors. "Me doctor, you nurse." Thank God times have changed with the ascension of female physicians.

Although they shared many stories, Grace found it strange that Emma never talked about her family. She knew she had a daughter who had children because she had alluded to the grandchildren, but unlike other parents, she never really talked about her own child. Grace got the feeling she was embarrassed or perhaps disappointed in how things had turned out for her children. As the years passed, they both maintained a good relationship until Emma retired from her work at the hospital. When the staff threw her a small retirement party, her family was in attendance. It was at that party that Grace Gallagher realized she knew Emma's daughter well. Doris Finley had changed back to her maiden name.

Jane Doe: Gutted.

Chapter 6 — Meat No More

A new decade for Doris meant the hope for a fresh start, both in her social life and her condition. Balancing single motherhood, two teenagers and several other surgeries had taken their toll. She had been to St. Francis so many times it seemed like her second home. Times had changed and with few religious staffing the hospital, but one nurse stuck in her mind. She always seemed to be working there. God, what was her name?

In the mid-eighties, Doris had an oophorectomy, the removal of her the ovaries and the fallopian tubes, usually done together as they share the same blood supply. Although these are relatively safe procedures, Doris' lack of luck continued its downward spiral. She suffered risks associated with these surgeries, including depression, decreased sex drive and memory problems.

In spite of her conditions, tonight was a night to celebrate. She was serious about this new guy, Gary Donovan, a gentleman in his mid-50s. Older meant stable, something she could desperately use a good dose of, since all the hospital visits put a strain on her financial resources. Even though she had a good law practice, surgeries cost money and so did teenagers. She met Gary, himself divorced, at the courthouse where he was undergoing a custody battle for his only child. While it was ugly, Gary remained a gentleman throughout the ordeal, rare for these court spectacles.

Tonight they were celebrating at Halverson's Chop House, a very upscale eatery, especially for Athens, Ohio. They had talked about going to Cleveland, but didn't want to make the two hour drive on New Year's Eve.

The couple started out with drinks, a dry martini for him and a Manhattan for her, and one of her favorite hors d'oeuvres, mushroom

Jane Doe: Gutted.

polenta on toasted garlic points. The conversation was casual, a little about his work in savings and loan, and very little about hers. She was in the middle of a very tough case and legally couldn't discuss it.

Gary motioned to the server, "I'll have another ... Doris?"

"Sure, why not. It's New Year's Eve," she replied.

"I've been dying to try this place out. The guys at the bank said the steaks are out of this world."

"Great. I haven't had steak in ages. With the kids' schedule and mine, fast food seems to be the norm these days."

As the round of drinks arrived, Gary raised his glass in a toast as Doris joined him.

"To your health," he smiled.

"To a new decade of health," she emphasized.

For a small city, Halverson's put on quite a spread. The steak was perfection, hers rare, and the accompanying sides, twice-baked garlic potatoes, asparagus tips in Cabot cheese sauce were savored along with the conversation. Dessert had been ordered, a caramel soufflé, when Doris squirmed with sudden discomfort.

The initial pain appeared as a persistent dull ache under her ribcage. As the dessert arrived, the discomfort suddenly escalated into a sharp, jabbing pain. Doris quickly excused herself and barely made it to the ladies room where she vomited profusely into the sink. After returning to the table to an alarmed Gary, her face a bit ashen, he expressed concern.

"Are you okay? Was it the food?" he asked.

"I'm not sure. You had the same thing. Maybe I just ate too fast."

Once again, she felt the urgent need to retreat to the restroom and this time it necessitated a toilet. The intense diarrhea was like nothing she had ever experienced. On exiting the restroom, she passed out.

The end of a perfect date.

Jane Doe: Gutted.

St. Francis was staffed for an always-busy New Year's Eve. The nurses and doctors were accustomed to alcohol poisonings, car accidents and, being a small city, the occasional gunshot patients.

The radio alerted the desk to an incoming transmission.

"Forty year old, white female, intense vomiting, diarrhea and abdominal pain ... conscious and responsive ... ETA six minutes," and the radio bleeped silent.

Personnel in the E.R. had changed over the years. The only familiar face was Nurse Grace Gallagher, now 54 and still working despite repeated warnings from annoyed doctors. The only thing that really saved her ass up to now was being superb at her job.

Dr. Wilson was a smart, bland, no-bedside-manner physician. Not Grace's favorite. No surprise.

As Doris was wheeled into the E.R. and into a waiting bay, Nurse Gallagher again winced at seeing her special patient in such pain. Wilson pulled and prodded at Doris, she cried out in pain and moaned.

"Oh my God, that hurts!"

And as Grace feared and like many doctors, Wilson arrived at the much too comfortable conclusion.

"It's her gallbladder. Notify the O.R. she'll need a cholecystectomy stat," he barked.

Once again, Doris was going under the knife. She wondered if it would be different with a female doctor. Would they be less likely to jump to the same conclusion or was it too late to save her gallbladder?

Diet, Grace thought almost out loud, "Monkeys don't get gallstones because they are vegan." Understanding we don't swing from trees, we could still learn that increasing fiber is an absolute. More fruit, vegetables, whole grains and lentils should be introduced into the diet at a younger age. And eat the good fruits: apples, figs, prunes, berries and

Jane Doe: Gutted.

apricots, to name a few. Fish containing Omega-3, also helps prevent cholesterol build-up.

The gallbladder produces bile that breaks down fats. Unfortunately, those include meat, ice cream, French fries, pizza and God forbid, movie theater buttered popcorn. When the gallbladder is removed, 60% of the patients return to a relatively normal intestinal health. For others like Doris, such was not the case. The body was still producing bile, but the regulator had been removed. Extreme bloating and gas was her new normal along with immediate bathroom visits after each meal. Constant abdominal pain was also a new reality.

She would soon realize she could never digest meat ever again, forcing her into a vegetarian diet. Ironically enough, this type of diet could have changed the downward spiral her body had been on.

Jane Doe: Gutted.

Chapter 7 — The Inquisition

In Grace Gallagher's mind, she had been called to the principal's office, Mother Ignatius, a Sister of no Mercy.

In reality, the years of challenging the authority of doctors she worked for had come back to haunt her. Dr. Wilson's last entry into Grace's file had prompted this meeting. Present in the room were the Medical Executive Committee consisting of Dr. Wilson; the Director of Nursing, Miss Rosemarie Carpenter; from Human Resources, Mr. Harold Thigpen; and the Hospital Administrator, Mr. Terrence Fitzgerald.

Miss Carpenter was the first to speak since her job as Director of Nursing was the supervision and administration of all the nurses at St. Francis. Being a nurse herself, she understood the importance of the position yet the repeated insubordination noted in Grace Gallagher's file demanded a resolution.

"The reasons we called you here today were presented to you in writing on January 23rd," she droned on as she introduced the others on the panel.

Although Grace was listening, she was surprised that this day hadn't come sooner. In fact, she had already planned for her "retirement" from St. Francis and recently purchased a tiny little gift shop in the local mall.

"Mr. Thigpen?" Miss Carpenter finished and he cleared his throat.

"We all are in agreement that your work is exemplary, but..."

Blah, blah, blah. You're a great nurse, but you're uncensored opinions have been a constant problem. Grace had heard this diatribe many times before.

What she wanted to tell them and would never get the chance, is there was a good reason for her obstinance. Nurturing a healthy lifestyle in children and maintaining that through their adult life gets you a free

Jane Doe: Gutted.

pass out of surgery. It's a long sentence for a simple reality: Eat better, live longer.

I had been lucky enough to be enlightened by the fact that through a healthy diet, vitamin supplements and moderate exercise, many diseases can be avoided. The human body is a machine, and like all machines, it needs to be properly maintained and well-oiled. Obesity, diabetes, cancer, strokes and heart attacks can be prevented altogether. I am not trying to put St. Francis out of business. It is filled with brilliant doctors and nurses who literally work miracles every day. Surgery is the last chance miracle. This medical procedure is the plumber, the electrician and the carpenter for a broken body. Look at all of the lives it saves.

But my whole mantra all along has been: How much better would it be if we didn't have to get to this Hail Mary pass? Obviously, I could have been handled it better, but unfortunately as a nurse I was not in an influential position. By the time I had the chance to interact with the patient, typically it was too late. Look at poor Doris. I have seen her from a baby through mid-life and fear for her well-being.

"As of February first," Thigpen pontificated, "You will no longer be on-staff at St. Francis Memorial Hospital. Thank you for your time and service." He looked around the room. "Is there anything else?" Everyone remained silent. They all rose and shuffled out with Dr. Wilson being the last one out, puzzled by Grace's serene look.

Grace had no regrets for her actions.

Jane Doe: Gutted.

Chapter 8 — Things Forgot

Doris was about to reach a milestone. She liked to call it "59.95 plus tax." She was turning sixty. The last twenty years of her life had consisted of events, good and bad, and her mother, Emma, had passed and her sister, Louise, had become quite estranged. Doris' kids, both married, were in touch sporadically, usually when the news was not good. Doris still worshipped Tony and was faithful to his memory. She considered it a privilege to have been able to love and be loved like that, even if their love was a secret and not sanctified by marriage, something they had planned on.

Basically, the last decade had been used to build her law practice, which flourished.

Medically, she had been fairly stable and her only concern was her propensity for using notes. Sticky notes. Everywhere. Be it a grocery list or the dry cleaner to detailed instructions on case law for her paralegal to research. Her mind seemed to be playing tricks on her and, like we all do, she chalked it up to aging.

Today was a particularly important day and she could barely make it out the door. The Law Offices of Finley & McAfee were scheduled to argue a case in the Court of Appeals, 11th Appellate District in Ashtabula County, Ohio. Her own County of Athens was some four hours away from Ashtabula. This case had been brought to the firm by a desperate mother eager to overturn a sexual predator evaluation filed on her son.

Doris' partner, David McAfee, was in court on a case in Athens, so it fell to Doris to make the long trek. They had been preparing for this case for months and she had hoped David would be able to argue before the court.

Doris reviewed her mental checklist and the assortment of sticky notes on the dashboard. She popped in a Harry Connick Jr. CD and sped

Jane Doe: Gutted.

off toward the Interstate highway. Two hours into the trip, she remembered she forgot her cellphone, note six on the dashboard. Seemingly when a note had been there for a while, it seemingly vanished from her psyche. Doris arrived at the courthouse just in time to grab a cup of coffee with the defendant's mother at a small kiosk in front of the courthouse.

Judge Burton Pierce, an avuncular man, had been sitting on the bench for twenty-five years. He was known to be fair, but a stickler for the letter of the law.

At the stroke of ten, the proceedings started.

"All rise. Judge Burton Pierce presiding. The State of Ohio versus Richard Duane White, case number 2002-D-0088," droned the Bailiff.

Doris took a deep breath, knowing she was well prepared, but even after all these years, hated performing in court.

In evidence was the testimony of the "FPCONO," Lawrence Halbert, the Executive Director of the Forensic Psychiatric Center of Northeast Ohio. Halbert stated that the appellant was given an MMPI test and that the appellant had extremely high scores on the psychopathic deviant scale showing characteristics of an anti-social personality disorder. Also, since the appellant had prior sex offense convictions using extreme force and cruelty, there was indeed a pattern of anti-social behavior.

As Doris rose to rebut this testimony, she simply forgot the name of her client. Normally, she would glance down at her notes on the defense table, but she was paralyzed in her panic.

She simply forgot the name of her client.

Unfortunately, for Doris, there was nothing simple about it. Forces unknown to her had been at work in her body. A body that had been ravaged by years of medical responses that had left her with a compromised immune system.

"Your honor, if I may have a short recess?" Doris pleaded.

Jane Doe: Gutted.

The smile on Judge Pierce's face turned to a frown as proceedings had just started. He banged the gavel.

"The court will recess for ten minutes."

Doris fled to the restroom to catch her breath. She seemed overly flushed and extremely winded. Consciously, she had no idea what was happening, but subconsciously she knew. It had been a slow process, seemingly over the last five years, but this had probably been ten years in the making.

Doris Finley looked in the mirror.

"You need to stop kidding yourself. You know what's happening and you have to stop it." She splashed her face with cold water and spoke to herself once again in a measured tone, "His name is Richard Duane White and you are his lawyer."

She sighed in relief.

Jane Doe: Gutted.

Chapter 9 — Reunion

Dr. Eammon checked the pupils of Grace Gallagher's eyes as Nurse Hernandez attended to the cut on her head.

"It's a slight laceration, relatively shallow with a brief loss of consciousness," Grace surmised.

"Thank you doctor ..."

"Nurse Gallagher. Worked in this E.R. for over thirty years." Hernandez chuckled.

Dr. Eammon had none of this, "Do you know today's date?"

"December nineteen, twenty thirteen."

"And the president?"

Grace became her old self and toys with the ill-mannered doctor.

"Well, it should have been Hillary," she smiled, "but I believe it's still Mr. Obama. I like him, he just not a woman."

Dr. Eammon continued with his curt bedside manner.

"She's fine, just stitch her up," as he snapped off his gloves and dropped them to the floor as he left the bay.

She thought to herself, "One of those." She turned to Hernandez.

"Who pissed in his corn flakes this morning?"

Hernandez sized up Grace before he answered.

"Take your pick. You know the type. The attending with attitude."

She reads his name tag.

"Hernandez, who's heading up the E.R. today?"

"Dr. Chip Fitzgerald. He's in the next room with the patient that arrived with you. They're in the process of identifying her."

"Presenting in a state of dementia?"

"Yes," he paused, knowing he should not have discussed another patient.

"Could you call Dr. Fitzgerald in here please?"

Jane Doe: Gutted.

Confused, Hernandez hesitated.

"I have information on the patient."

He breathed a sigh of relief as he left to get Dr. Fitzgerald.

Grace reposed on the table reviewing the events of the morning in her mind. With her work at Heavenly Detours in the last twenty years, she had little time to think about her days at St. Francis. She had seen hundreds of patients, but for some reason, Doris Finley had always stuck in her mind.

The whoosh of the curtain in the bay snapped her back to reality.

"Hello, Miss Gallagher."

The ambience of the entire room changed with three simple words. If this was Chip Fitzgerald, she planned on a return to nursing! The six-two, tanned, blond, blue-eyed professional at the foot of the bed looked out of place in scrubs. Better he stood in front of a camera starring in his own TV series. God help us all if he was nice, too.

He eased around to her bedside.

"Johnny said you had some information on my patient that you'd like to share," he smiled.

Perfect teeth, perfect smile. Perfection.

"Her name is Doris Finley," Grace began, "And her medical path to today has been varied and unfortunate for her. Should I continue?"

He laid his hand on her hand, "I understand, we're both professionals here, so please fill me in."

Grace succinctly outlined Doris' medical history and of her own relationship with her.

Chip again flashed those perfect teeth, "So, you were a rebel."

"And proud of it," Grace said.

"I hear you."

With those three words, she knew he was of a like mind and kindred spirit.

"Level with me, Dr. Fitzgerald."

Jane Doe: Gutted.

"Chip, please."

"What kind of a name is Chip?"

"Nickname, chip off the old block. Dad is head of surgery at Johns Hopkins."

"So, it's in your blood?"

"Well, more of a transfusion. I wanted to be carpenter, good with my hands."

"Oh that must be one of your best lines."

They both laughed.

"What happened?"

Without hesitation, "It was a trade-off. They accepted my lifestyle and I accepted their vocation."

"So, back to your patient, Chip. In what stage of dementia is she?"

"I am not sure at this point, I can only assess what I see. Was she violent?"

"Combative."

"Sorry to say, but the police have been called," he advised.

"I was hoping that wouldn't happen, I certainly won't press charges."

"I assume then it will be a disorderly conduct charge."

Dr. Fitzgerald proceeded to examine Grace's cut.

"Hernandez did a good job with these and not much will show after the stitches come out."

"I won't worry, my beauty pageant days are over."

He laughed, "Sorry you're still not here, Grace. You'd fit in here perfectly."

"Do you have a good consult in mind for Doris?" Grace asked.

"In fact, I do. And you'd love her. A doctor with a sense of humor and a good head on her shoulders."

Jane Doe: Gutted.

Jane Doe: Gutted.

Chapter 10 — Evaluation

Doris Finley found herself at the door of a small, boutique clinic operated by Dr. Berta Briones & Associates. She had worked hard to make her appearance as presentable as possible and she felt lucky today was a good day. Her daughter, Marci, had helped her with wardrobe, jewelry and she hardly needed her GPS to find the location.

With great trepidation, she climbed the steps past the potted peonies to ring the doorbell.

Denise greeted her at the door, "Hello, Miss Finley, I'm Denise Cloutier, Dr. Briones' assistant. Come in, we've been expecting you."

She ushered Doris past a waiting room directly into a smartly furnished sea foam green office.

"Would you care for some tea or bottled water to drink?" Denise asked.

"Water would be lovely," Doris smiled.

Doris sat apprehensively, as if she was waiting for sentencing to come down from the court. She has researched her condition on her own and realized the situation had deteriorated. She had been appalled at her behavior at Heaven's Detours at the Springfield Mall. She was indebted to Grace Gallagher for not pressing charges.

Dr. Berta Briones was a maverick in her field, combining traditional medicine with preventative and holistic elements to her patients' regime. Loathing a lab coat, she often dressed in business casual, stepping off the pages Chico's Fall Collection.

"Good of you to come, Doris. Did you want something to drink?" she asked.

"Denise is getting me water."

"Good, good," as Dr. Briones sat in the winged chair across form Doris.

Jane Doe: Gutted.

"I'll be honest, being in the legal profession, I'm a get-to-it kind of person."

"Then we will get along perfectly," the doctor smiled.

"And I've done a lot of my own research," Doris said.

In one breath, Dr. Briones sized up the patient before her and realized a direct approach was the best.

"You have dementia and we are here today to find out what stage you're in. This is a state that causes a loss of mental function, thinking, memory, and often reasoning. While dementia is not actually a disease per se, it is a group of symptoms that are caused by other conditions. Substance abuse?"

"Never," Doris replied.

"Good, good. Including prescription meds?"

"Never abused."

"And finally, depression?"

Doris thought a moment, "After my second child, yes. And I feel it contributed to the cause of my divorce."

"In a way, this may sound strange, but I'm glad to hear that."

Doris was indeed surprised.

"I don't mean the divorce part, I mean the depression, it's easier to treat. With hormone and vitamin supplements, we can try to stall the dementia."

"Will this turn into Alzheimer's?" Doris feared.

"Common misconception, Alzheimer's may be a cause of the dementia as with many other causes. Dementia is the spectrum into which Alzheimer's may fit as a cause."

"Okay, now I understand," she sighed.

"Alzheimer's is a buzzword that in its own reality is horrifying, but as I said, there may be other causes," the doctor continued, "Your medical history? Any kidney, liver or lung disease?"

Jane Doe: Gutted.

"Appendectomy, hysterectomy, oophorectomy and cholecystectomy," Doris recounted.

"So, no appendix, no uterus, no ovaries and no gallbladder. I guess we're lucky they left you with a brain."

"I guess that's the next thing to go," Doris chuckled.

"That sense of humor and a healthier plan of attack is going to improve your mental functioning, although I cannot make any promises. There are not enough studies to be able to give you any statistics.

"This is a lifestyle change, but we're at a crossroads here. You have had some very bad days, correct?"

Doris sat quietly, reflecting on the event at the Springfield Mall. That was one of the worst episodes, but there were others that came very close. Doris realized she had lost complete days where she remembered nothing and she assumed on those days she did not know who she was.

"My program is not a miracle pill, sorry," Dr. Briones emphasized.

"It's a lot to take in," Doris said.

Dr. Briones beamed with an effervescent smile, "I know it is," she took a deep breath before beginning a mini-history of cause and effect for Doris' condition.

"We need to do damage control. We need to mitigate all the injustices your body has been subjected to over the years. The organs in our bodies are there for a reason. The appendix helps produce probiotics, the good bacteria that keep our gut in balance. The gut is called the second brain because it produces lots of neurotransmitters needed for brain function. Your poor diet led you to suffer from digestive problems that ended up with your appendix inflamed and needing to come out, which prevented you from dying. Your gallbladder, a major detoxification organ, got full of gallstones due to multiple reasons. High cholesterol comes from either diet or from lack of hormones produced by the ovaries or testicles. A result is the liver trying to produce more cholesterol, causing the adrenals to make more hormones. Then, from stasis of the

Jane Doe: Gutted.

gallbladder, which means there are things that make the gallbladder contract, such as chewing. When losing weight rapidly, pregnancy or liquid diets, the gallbladder does not contract for long periods of time. The stones, therefore, get bigger and one day you eat something that makes the gallbladder contract, ending with a stone stuck in the GB duct. The GB duct bursts or gets infected, needing to come out. Too late. Your uterus which you lost due to perimenopause, caused progesterone levels to drop. Unfortunately, the standard of care does not include hormone optimization. You either get an ablation, burn the lining of the uterus that bleeds, or get the entire uterus is removed. Either way, you do not receive treatment for the cause of the bleeding or progesterone deficiency, and that is a brain health essential hormone. Needless to say, hormones are not just for reproducing, they act in the brain to keep it functioning properly. Of course, balance is the key."

"Understood," Doris interjected.

"There are numerous case reports where people's brain activity have improved with mild hyperbaric oxygen therapy, neurofeedback and good quality supplements such as IV phosphatidyl choline, B vitamins, vinpocetine, huperzine and ginkgo biloba. Also, there's hormone optimization, healthy diet and exercise. In a healthy diet, I'd include juicing, because of the ability to remove nutrients from fruits and vegetables, resulting in easier digestion. Do your research in buying a juicer, not all extract at the same degree of efficiency. Also, wheat grass juicing, a good quality chlorella supplementation for detoxification and for nutritional support. We will do a nutritional evaluation to see your nutrient deficiencies and target them, a toxicology evaluation, a hormonal evaluation, a physical fitness evaluation and, of course, cognitive baseline evaluation. My program is a comprehensive mind-body evaluation with the goal of restoring more youthful levels of functioning not only for the mind but for the body and spirit.

Doris struggled to digest all the information.

Jane Doe: Gutted.

"When do we start therapy?" she said affirmatively.

"That's the spirit I was banking on."

As Doris left to make further appointments for dieticians with Denise, the doctor reflected on the file in front of her. Doris Finley, early sixties and on the scale of the seven stages of dementia, was presumed to be at stage four, moderately cognitive decline.

There is a lot of evidence about preventing the onset of dementia for about eight years following Dr. Amen's plan.

Unfortunately, there is little evidence on reversing dementia. Dr. Briones felt her regime for the patient would stall the inevitable. Maybe, with luck and new therapies being discovered every day, there would be renewed hope for Doris Finley.

Jane Doe: Gutted.

Epilogue

Quoting Dr. Daniel Amen on the Encyclopedia of Clinical Antiaging Medicine and Regenerative Biomedical Technologies - 2012, "Alzheimer's Disease and Related Disorders," (ADRD) an acronym used to define a group of diseases that have one thing in common, commonality being a course of mild cognitive impairment (MCI) or dementia. Dementia is a progressive condition with two or more impairments in mental skills that interfere with a person's ability to function in his usual manner in his social, family, personal or professional life. A delay in diagnosis and treatment leads to less effective results.

Alzheimer's disease (AD) begins an average of 30 years before the first symptoms. Half of U.S. families have a member with Alzheimer's disease. The chance of developing AD doubles every five years after the age of 65. By age 85, there is a 50% chance of developing AD. The average cost to the family is $200,000-$400,000 per AD relative over the 8-10 year course of the disease. More devastating is the severe psychological and social pain that families suffer.

The remarkable medical and scientific advances today allow the benefit of prevention through delay of an average of six years cutting the risk of ADRD by up to 50%.

Prevention through delay is useful in lessening the disability that occurs with many diseases of aging. By age 40, humans have fulfilled their evolutionary purpose of perpetuating the species. After that, the daily repair to the cells of brain and body can no longer keep up with the ongoing damage and function begins to decline. Add that to the loss of vital organs involved in digestion, detoxification and absorption of nutrients and the stresses of surgical procedures and post-operative recovery without addressing the underlying shut down of hormone production, such as progesterone, that not only works in the uterus but all over the body, including the brain.

"Jane Doe 2: Gutted," is a call to reviewing the mindset of removing organs when the body malfunctions and not addressing the underlying problems also affect the brain.

The body continues to malfunction despite the removal of the organ because the underlying problem has not been addressed. For example, the appendix is removed, but the underlying unhealthy gut remains Now, the gut is the second "brain" as it produces large amounts

Jane Doe: Gutted.

of neurotransmitters that work in the cerebral brain. Then a gallbladder is removed. Problem being, the gallbladder is a major detoxification organ. So, what happens to the toxins and the lifestyle that led to the gallbladder's removal? What do toxins do to the brain?

Following the surgical path for an average woman, the uterus is removed, although now with the advent of uterine ablation techniques the organ is preserved, yet neither procedure treats the underlying problem, progesterone deficiency.

Progesterone is a major neuroprotective hormone, so what happens to their brains long-term?

While there is more and more evidence that the brain can be regenerated with the use of hyperbaric therapy, stem cells, neurofeedback, nutrition, diet and hormones, the best strategy is still prevention. No one explains this better than my friend, Dr. Daniel Amen in many of his books. He advocates avoiding brain injuries by eating healthy, daily exercise, avoiding stress and toxic relationships. He also advises in thinking positive, sleeping well, including being treated for sleep disorders. We should avoid toxins; detoxify, breathe healthy air, consume supplements, get bio-identical hormones restored and challenge the brain with new hobbies, brain games and new interests.

A great mind is a very sad thing to lose.

But so is an appendix, a gallbladder and the uterus.

To a healthy and wholesome life!

Cheers!
Dr. Liam A. Briones
Medical Rejuvenation Institute
Twitter: @myrejuv
FB: @rejuvme
Web: www.medicalrejuvenationinstitute.com

Jane Doe: Gutted.

References and commentary.

1. Dietary Induction of cholesterol gallstones in the owl monkey: preliminary findings in a new animal model. Pekow CA, Weller RE, Schulte SJ, Lee SP.
   Feeding the owl monkey a high cholesterol diet leads to gallstones. A compelling study that sheds light into human gallstone prevention. These monkeys eat a vegan diet under natural conditions and do not get gallstones unless fed high cholesterol diet. Their biliary system is similar to that of humans.
2. Allen et al. Gallbladder Disease. Pathophysiology, Diagnosis and Treatment. US Pharmacist. 2013; 38(3):33-41
3. Weil Integrative Oncology, 2009
4. Pizzorno, et al. Text Book of Natural Medicine. 2013. P. 1388-1394
   Cruciferous vegetables may play a significant role in cancer prevention (high intake of broccoli, cauliflower, cabbage, kale, bok choy, Brussels sprouts, radish and various mustards has been associated with decreased cancer risk. Crucifers have high content of glucosinolates and their hydrolysis products, isothiocyanates, protect against carcinogenesis. Crucifers also contain flavonoids, polyphenols, vitamins, fiber and pigments that may have anticancer ax. Their most important mechanism is that they may inhibit phase I enzymes which can activate carcinogen metabolites and they induce phase II enzymes, such as glutathione transferase enzymes, which enhance carcinogen detoxification.
   Chemopreventive agents include vitamins, minerals, phytochemicals and synthetic compounds. The most promising right now include antioxidant hormone modulating or antiinfl biological.
5. Takahashi et al. H. Pilory infection is positively associated with asymptomatic gallstones: a large scale cross sectional study in Japan. J Gastroenterol. 2013 Jun (Epub ahead of print).
   4.74% of asymptomatic males and 4.11% of asymptomatic females were found to have gallstones by Ultrasound. In this study they found that H. Pillory infection was associated with gallstones and that H. Pillory eradication may lead to prevention of gallstones.
6. Banim, et al. The etiology of symptomatic gallstones quantification of the effects of obesity, alcohol and serum lipids on risk.

Jane Doe: Gutted.

Epidemiological and biomarker data from a UK prospective cohort study. J. Gastroenterol Hepatol 2011 Aug;23(8):733-40. A study of 25,639 men and women aged 40-74 years were enrolled and monitored for 14 years for symptomatic gallstones. Symptomatic gallstones developed in 296 people of which 67.9% were women. For every unit of alcohol consumed there was a 3% reduction in risk in men but not women. Increased HDL also decreased the risk in men and also in women. Increased body mass index (BMI) was also correlated with increased risk. 38% of incident cases of gallstones were associated with BMI above 25. Serum Triglycerides levels increased risk in both as well.

7. Walcher, et al. The effect of alcohol, tobacco and caffeine consumption and vegetarian diet on gallstone prevalence. Eur J Gastroenterol Hepatol. 2010 Nov;22(11):1345-51. A cohort of 2417 individuals underwent US exam. The prevalence was 8% of gallstones. Age, female sex, obesity and positive family history were confirmed as risk factors.

Tobacco and caffeine consumption and vegan diet did not have any effect on Gallstone prevalence. A protective effect against gallstone was shown for alcohol consumption.

The treatments of asymptomatic gallstones include oral bile acids such as chenodeoxycholic acid (chenodiol) and ursodeoxycholic acid (ursodiol). The first one has too many side effects so the second one ursodiol is the one used more often. Symptom relief occurs in 3-6 weeks and results may take 6-24 months. (8-10mg/kg/day divided in 2-3 doses) and it is used to prevent gallstones during periods of rapid weight loss (diets or bariatric surgery) in doses of 300mg twice a day. Commons side effects include: Headache, dizziness, diarrhea, constipation, dyspepsia, nausea, vomiting, back pain, upper respiratory tract infection.

8. Portincasa, et al. Therapy of gallstone disease: What it was, what it is, what it will be. World J. Gastrointest Pharmacol Ther 2012 Apr 6; 3(2):7-20

Cholesterol lowering drugs which inhibit cholesterol synthesis (statins) or drugs that reduce intestinal cholesterol absorption (ezetimibe) or drugs acting on specific nuclear receptors involved in cholesterol and bile acid homeostasis might be proposed as additional approaches for treating cholesterol gallstones.

Non genetic risk factors for gallbladder stones; age, female, hi cl, lo fiber diet, high cholesterol diet , dietary glycemic load, obesity,

Jane Doe: Gutted.

physical inactivity, rapid weight loss/surgery for obesity, total gastrectomy with lymph node dissection, spinal cord injury, infections such as enterohepatic helicobacter sp, malaria and biliary strictures, Drugs: estrogens, calcineurin inhibitors, fibrates, octreotide, ceftriaxone. Total parenteral nutiriton, duodenal diverticulum, extended ileal resection (black pigment stones) vitb12/folate deficient diet (black stones) pancreatic insufficiency, cholangitis (brown pigment bile duct stones)

9. Robins Basic Pathology-9th Edition. Kumar, Abas, Aster. Chapter 14: Oral cavity and Gastrointestinal tract. Chapter 15: Liver, Gallbladder and Biliarty Tract. Chapter 18: Female genital system and Breast.
10. Ingelsson E, Lundholm C, Johansson ALV, and Altman D. Hysterectomy and risk of cardiovascular disease: a population based cohort study. *Eur Heart J* 2010; DOI:10.1093/eurheartj/ehq477. This study found a correlation between hysterectomy and cardiovascular disease in women, but to what degree was the underlying hormonal imbalances the primary cause? The authors concluded : The underlying mechanism may be that hysterectomy interferes with ovarian blood flow and may result in premature ovarian failure and hormone-related effects on the vascular bed.
11. HRT for Chronic Disease Prevention: Jury Is Still Out CME/CE News Author: Larry Hand, CME Author: Charles P. Vega, MD, FAAFP This is a review of the JAMA article *JAMA*. 2013;310:1349-1350, 1353-1368. They showed an increase in cardiovascular disease with hormone replacement in older women, but the big caveat is that they used synthetic estrogens and progesterone that the body identifies as foreing and reacts to them.
12. T. Hertoghe, Hormone Handbook, 2nd edition, International Medical books, www.imbooks.info.
13. The Gerson Therapy: The proven nutritional program for cancer and other illnesses. –Gerson and Walker, DPM.
14. Unleash the power of the female brain: supercharging yours for better health, energy, mood and sex. Dr. Daniel G. Amen -2012
15. Use your brain to change your age. Dr. Daniel G. Amen
16. The Amen solution: The Brain Healthy way to loose weight and keep it off. –Dr. Daniel G. Amen
17. Change your brain, change your Body: Use your brain to keep the body that you have always wanted. Dr. Daniel G. Amen.
18. Magnificent mind at any age. Dr. Daniel G. Amen.

Jane Doe: Gutted.

19. Change your brain change your life: a breakthrough program for conquering anxiety, depression, obsessiveness, anger and impulsiveness. –Dr. Daniel G. Amen.
20. Textbook of Nutrient Therapy-The International evidence based Medical textbook on Nutritional Therapies- Hertoghe et al. – International Medical Books.
21. Textbook of Lifespan and Anti-Aging Medicine: How to make healthy people healthier and live longer-Herthoge et al. –International Medical Books.
22. The wisdom and healing power of whole foods: The ultimate handbook for using whole foods and life style changes to bolster your body's ability to repair and regulate itself. –Patrick Quillin, PhD, RD, CNS.
23. Bacteria for breakfast: Probiotics for good health. Kelly Dowhower Karpa, PhD, RPh
24. Exitotoxins: The taste that kills. Russel L Blaylock MD.
25. Encyclopedia of clinical Anti-Aging Medicine & Regenerative Biomedical Technologies.-Klatz, Goldman et al.
26. Hyperbaric Oxygen for Neurological Disorders. John H. Shang MD, PhD et al.

Jane Doe: Gutted.

About the Author

Dr. Briones is a physician entrepreneur, scientist and life long learner who is interested in becoming the best healer that he can be and after he realized that he can't do it without the help of his patients he begun the Jane Doe series to empower his patients with knowledge to direct their life styles into a healthy future.

Dr. Briones is ABIM certified in Internal Medicine, Pulmonary and Critical Care , Board Certified by the American Academy of Sleep Medicine and by the American Board of Anti-Aging and Regenerative Medicine. He completed the advanced fellowship training at the A4M and the Integrative Cancer Fellowship in 2013. He graduated from the University of Tennessee Physician Executive MBA program in 2002.